BLANSHARD AND BLANSHARD

UNFU*K
YOURSELVES

LOVE-CHANGING MAGIC. HOW TO STOP
MESSING UP RELATIONSHIPS, SO YOU
CAN SKIP ARGUMENTS, BE HAPPIER,
SPARK LOVE, AND STAY TWOGETHER
FOREVER

PAGE ADDIE PRESS
UNITED KINGDOM. AUSTRALIA

Published 2017 by Page Addie Press. United Kingdom, Australia.
Unfu*k Yourselves. Love-changing magic. How to stop messing up relationships so
you can skip arguments, be happier, spark love, and
stay twogether forever
Copyright© All rights reserved Blanshard & Blanshard

A CIP record for this book is available from the British Library,
and Australian Library.
ISBN: 978-064695810-1 paperback.
BIC Subject category VS: 1. Self-Help - Personal Transformation - relationship 2.
Self-Help - Motivational. 3. Health Fitness & Dieting - Mental Health - happiness.
4. Self-Help - Interpersonal Relations - couples. 5. Self-Help - Success - couples.
6. Humour & Entertainment - Humour - parodies. 7. Humour & Entertainment -
Humour - Self-Help - Psychology.

CONTENT

Unfu*k Yourselves!

Relationships don't fuck themselves up. They are never fucked to begin with or we wouldn't be in them. It takes us to fuck them. It happens in the micro moments: relationships start to get a little fucked up when we miss each other's clues or send and receive confusing signals; they get more fucked when we talk but don't communicate. They get really fucked when we let problems emerge as arguments; or your partner doesn't listen or validate your feelings, making you feel unloved. It's just fucked! Relationships sometimes get so fucked up, we can't wait to walk away from the mess.

Do you make up more than you make out?

It didn't use to be like this! How did this happen?

5

Is Love A Four Letter Word?

Do you remember when you first met you called each other cutesie nicknames like baby, lover, sweetheart? Those honey names. Even if you promised you'd never give each other sappy names, it just happened. So if 'Angel' made you sound like a shape-shifter or some kind of a supernatural being, it didn't matter. It wasn't about the name was it - big guy, hottie, babydoll, the names that made single friends' eyes roll. Everything you did for each other seemed so right.

So, what about names you call each other now? Are any built around four letter words like:

fU¢* ÿðU!

There's a saying:

*In the **first year** of a relationship, one partner listens to the other, in the **second year** of a relationship, the other partner listens, in the **third year**, the neighbors listen to them both and they're hearing a four-letter word, and it isn't love.*

Have you ever thought to yourself (even once or a hundred times) Fu*k you! What the hell am I doing with you? Why don't I pack my bags and get out? My mother was probably right! There must be someone better. What did I ever see in you? I must have been out of my mind!

There's no place for this kind of thinking in a long term loving relationship. So sooner or later, you'll both have to sort your issues out, because this constant negative attitude just won't work out. And you know, that unless you can make this work, you'll end up leaving a bad relationship or worse staying in one. If you don't sort it out, you'll be back looking for the 'perfect' partner again. Yet, the more partners you spend time with, the harder it is to experience love, long term.

It's logical unless you address the core of the issues, the same problems will cause the same issues, no matter what relationship you are in. And at this rate, you'll be pushing up blooming daisies instead of holding a bunch of long stem red roses in your hands.

Honestly, ask yourself this question. Is this relationship almost a statistic? Could it become one? Have you both become jaded enough to secretly believe that any long term relationship is too hard to achieve and impossible to obtain? It comes down to one big comparison: how things are right now, compared to how things were when you first met and spent time together.

When you're singleton, you make all your own

decisions and you work out your own patterns on how you're doin' life. Life is as complex and simple as you choose. Then one day, someone special comes winging into your life. When you fall in love with someone the feeling is complete. Love is love is love. It's a wonderous infatuating feeling, beyond words. All of the kissing, cuddles, intimate and romantic times, adds into your life a whole love level. When that happens, you still do what you've always done but with the addition of spending time with the one you've fallen in love with. Then, because you are a couple, within this coupleness you start to add into the romantic mix, real-time joint decisions for the day to day lives you now share like: which restaurant for dinner, what groceries do we need, what movie, who's friend's place for dinner.

As life gets more complicated so do the decisions like: move in together?, paint the bedroom walls melon?, fancy goldfish or a suckermouth or swordtail?, black kitten, or rescue a puppy from the pound?

The longer you are together, the bigger the joint decisions like: the wedding, the baby, changing jobs, making career adjustments, child-rearing, location and relocation, buying the apartment, mortgages, savings, investments, vehicles, bills, expenses, budget, running the household, walking the dog, another baby, schools, clothes, in-laws, and vacations – you both want to go to the same place! The bigger the life decisions, the more complicated. So many decisions are made by agreeing with someone else on what you do. This is where all the communication, loss of personal freedom and identity issues, requirements for trust, honesty, openness, loving understanding, patience, tolerance, anger management, emotional I.Q., compromise, helping, giving, listening and talking things through, become very important. The complexity of communication from doin' life, in general, can become a hindrance to the easygoing, ongoing, exciting love experience you had when you first got together, because now more sophisticated communication is needed. More than you needed in the very beginning of your relationship when external demands were a whole lot less.

Out of all the people in the world, you chose to be with each other. That made for a beautiful beginning. The essential love you had in the early stages hasn't gone anywhere, it won't have gone away, it hasn't disappeared in a puff of proverbial smoke, love is still there, believe it! It's just that love becomes awfully dominated by the everyday complexity of living in a shared relationship. And if you're not careful, it turns into a hindrance to happiness when this translates to not feeling so much in love, and that translates to not being as much in love as you once were. It can become all so complicated that it gets completely fucked up and you lose the dynamics of love that got you together in the first place.

There are degrees of fu*kedness. It's when you keep adding fu*ked up stuff, to the already fu*ked up stuff, that the relationship gets really fu*ked up. You end up putting up with it all and accepting this as the new norm; criticizing each other for making your life miserable.

The problem isn't your relationship per se. It's the problems you've both embedded in the relationship: the trivia, the petty, the bitchy and the multiple misunderstandings. They force you to finger-point, say something sarcastic, feel contempt; whisper shitty retorts, like, "fuck off!" "fuck you!" "go fuck yourself!" Love-wrecking thoughts.

Of course, every personal relationship is different, but the key principles are the same. You have a bunch of fu*ked up stuff you've done, or said and continue to do and say. Bad stuff gets dumped into your relationship on a daily, weekly or monthly basis. It doesn't go anywhere of its own accord. The relationship is as messy as an unmade bed and as cluttered as a closet; crap mounts up at an alarming rate. You can't see it, but you can feel it and it doesn't feel good. It's relationship physics. What you put in, stays there, the good, the bad and crap.

Unfu*k Yourselves In 7 Days!

What if you could just unfuck yourselves? What if you could remove the crappy bits out of your relationship? You'd be so much more into each other, right? What if you could use fun to solve problems. You don't have to be comedy channel funny, but you can have fun resolving issues, together. Why not do just that? See all problems as:

'a wake-up call'

Whatever issues you have can be solved easily by understanding the issue and talking *twogether*. Some problems are easy to resolve. Not spending enough time together? Easy: make a date. There are other problems that take a while to sort, but every problem is fixable. First,

11

identify issues that are bugging you. The problems that replay themselves over and over in arguments. The ones that repeat like a belch. The ones that make up the burgeoning list of issues that never seem to go away.

There might be two or ten or twenty things you wish weren't problems in your relationship. You can't wish those away; it's not that easy, but you can sort each and every one, communicating with love, honesty, trust and respect. Respect your thoughts, respect your ability to do certain things on both sides, not one side.

Make a short list of these issues. When you identify a problem, look into it and discuss it. Look closely at it together, and be honest, you'll start to understand how attitudes, or what someone says or doesn't say, is making the issue stick. Each week, decide to work together on just one unresolved issue. After one week you may not have ironed out the issue completely, but you'll both recognize its pattern and gained a better understanding. By focusing on them, working things out, you'll improve your *twogetherness*. It's remarkable how in one week, most issues can become nonissues. Remember this, some issues took longer to develop, so some problems may take a week or two. However long it takes, it's all worth working on.

Sure, there are lots of reasons relationships can feel fucked-up – but that's no reason to give up. If you keep in mind, love is still there, it's just tied up at present! Because in your complicated lives;

P.S.
(Post Singleton)

-your needs and wants get inadvertently tangled up with a partner's need and wants – but that's not the end of it, all you have to do is unfuck yourselves. Think of unfucking yourselves as undoin' the fucked-up knots that happened as you built *The Big Life* together. As soon as you do this, more love flows back into your relationship. In a week you can go from doin' life together (with arguments thrown in) to doin' more living and loving together again!

Eraser

How will you know if an issue is erased? You simply won't notice it anymore. The problem that caused so much discord, just goes away of it's own accord. You'll never find yourselves arguing over it or thinking about it again. You simply looked at it, discussed it, without fighting about it; came up with a solution and practiced erasing the problem for a week. Then take another argument inducing problem and deal with it in the same way...a week later... it's no longer causing a problem. Two problems solved forever. Put in a few weeks of concentrated effort to unfu*k yourselves and you'll feel closer than you have in a long time.

When you have less conflict, you love more. When you fight less you have more energy to be loving; better friends and lovers. When you change the negative side of your relationship to the positive, you get so much more; more connected, more bonded, more intimate, more passion, more *twogether*.

Emotional Seltzer

Most relationship experts say ignore small issues and only look at big ones. We say, every issue creates effervescence; unresolved bubbles of negative energy, that surface again, and again, and again...every little bubble has the potential of creating explosive arguments. Fights! You have to stop the triggers of emotional flare-ups because unresolved issues take the lightness out of being together.

There is a huge difference between actually resolving issues and blindly arguing over them. The good news is without problems, there can't be growth in your relationship. What matters about problems is what you do with them.

The task is not to fix each other, not to change what your partner thinks or believes or their variables, but to gain understanding and greater respect for each other; the one you love and feel connected to, be they an idealist, success-orientated achiever, spontaneous enthusiast, powerful challenger, sensitive individualist, caring peacemaker, intense, funny, bold, ditzy, engaging, creative, entertaining... or all of the above, to love each other's quirks and foiables, uniqueness and awesome differences, the things that make them so special.

Intelligensia

You're both incredibly intelligent in real life. So if you bring issues out into the open, you're sure to resolve anything amicably.

"What issues?"
"You know... the problems!!?"
"I can't think that we have any real problems."
"Hey!?"

Wait a minute! There are no psychologists around here. Be honest. Only you two know which issues you need to resolve to make your relationship work. Break it down. What gets annoying? What makes you feel irritated? What makes you really pissed off.

You may have to admit you're wrong and that isn't easy. What is easy, is to find fault with your partner! No one's perfect and no one should point the finger. You know, you may be the one at fault. There will be times when you disagree, let it be and agree to disagree. No one has to be 'right', right?

Vampires

Problems that won't go away are like inglorious vampires. They suck the love out of your relationship before you know it; but once they are brought out into the open and see the light of day, problems fade away to nothing. You can make them vanish simply by making your partner aware that a problem you have talked about together, has arisen again. How can you do this effectively? You can do it by agreeing to say a short phrase linked to the problem that you both recognize and understand. Then every time the issue arises, just nail it by saying a specific phrase. Many of the chapter headings in this book are examples of problem phrases like:

'Acid Rain'
'P. K'
'Spinach'

Short phrase alerts allow one or both of you to immediately turn the situation around. Make up a bunch of your own sayings and you've created a relationship repertoire to identify problem issues.

A couple shared their phrase recently: "MTM". Now, we had no idea what MTM meant until they explained it. To that couple, it means one specific thing: you're being Mean To Me. A potent signal, one voiced, they both got completely. A way of saying, "I've had enough of this attitude. Be nice!' The phrase MTM acted as an argument diffuser and it worked a treat to stop them fighting.

When you make up a list of short phrases ahead of time, you create dynamic emotional shortcuts, so when you're out and about, you simply cut to it and help each other out when you need to.

Hear the word a few times and you'll see what is going on in the relationship, the emotions involved and patterns of behavior towards each other. You even find yourselves laughing about the facets of various emotions, imperfections, and flaws.

You'll fight less...laugh and love more.

Eggshells

The way you communicate affects the way your relationship is. So the first step in creating a long-term relationship is to get honest with yourself and each other; don't lie. It's not going to be easy. You know why? As human beings, we have a great capacity to lie, tell half-truths and be manipulative. A relationship is not a place to aerate your lies. If you lie to avoid confrontation, keep the peace or to get our own way, your partner won't be able to rely on you. If you hide things to protect yourself or to make your partner feel better, then your partner will get the feeling you're not being truthful, and sure enough, you're not.

Deception scrambles communication

it's the opposite of being open and up front with each other. Rather than hiding the grit of reality and putting up a fake false front, be honest. Tell it like it is. Your truth. That way you'll be a clear thinker, a straight thinker. Live authentically and be true to yourself.

Let go of treading eggshells around each other. Agree to do the opposite. Instead of hiding feelings to protect yourself, instead of resisting and covering up emotions that are painful, simply get in a habit of sitting *twogether* and talking more openly. Open up and allow your feelings to be known and shared. You'll find yourselves talking *twogether*, not at each other. As you listen to each other, you'll feel a shift in the direction of soul to soul love, immediately.

Once you share your interior life with your lover; discuss honestly how you really feel about things, you'll define your emotional authenticity and you'll both experience a greater intimacy. Once you cut the pretend crap, the love comes back. You'll discover new ways to relate to each other. Both verbally and non-verbally.

Eggshells

Don't tread eggshells around each other.

Make it a double yolker.

The Bad Patch

Is falling in love and staying in love with the same person forever, really possible?

Yes!

But how do you move past days where love is going to pieces and you have no idea why. You're arguing all the time. Ruminating in your own feelings:

"Do I really love him? Does he love me? This isn't going to last. We're not in sync. What's happening to us? We just don't get on anymore! Things have never been this bad before!"

You may fear that one of you is going to dump out of the relationship at any given moment. Hold on a minute. While this sounds really bad it doesn't mean the relationship is over. You're just going through a bad patch.

It's important to remember: relationships are rarely mergers of strengths melding into perfection. What you have in common is your ability to accommodate each other's differences. What makes you fit together is this: your curves and bumps happen to match someone else's bumps and curves. But at times it just doesn't fit. So expect and accept that you're going to have bad patches.

Everyone goes through hard times in relationships. It just means there are some issues that need to be worked out. While this is going on, it is important to keep in mind, that this situation, this moment in time, is not permanent. No matter how impossible it seems. Spend this uncomfortable time working it out and not freaking out. With patience and a desire to stay together, every issue can be solved or resolved within the relationship.

Rather than focusing on the bad patch, make an effort to shift negative energy that is enveloping you as a couple. You can do this by stopping and deciding to do one good thing together. Even if you don't feel like it. It's really important to redirect yourselves in a positive way. You've got to add good things. When you're back to sharing good times again; you'll realize that the bad patch was a necessary adjustment. You didn't walk out the door, you postponed rash reactions and calmed the f*** down, you stayed together and worked through it. The bad patch was a good thing because it was just what you needed to strengthen and move the relationship on.

There is a difference between a short term relationship and a long term relationship. In short term relationships partners walk out during bad patches. In long term relationships, they don't. If you want a relationship to last, you've got to... make it happen.

The Bad Patch

Commit to staying together.

Do something good together.

Do something good for each other.

Work through the bad patch.

Trust that you can revive your relationship.

Chocolate

Good things balance out negativity. If things aren't
good between you right now this is where something simple
like chocolate helps! Chocolate gets right to the heart
of pleasure, by increasing the feel-good brain chemical
serotonin. Chocolate promotes the brain chemistry of love.
It's hard to argue about that! A cup of hot chocolate and a
bunch of red roses too. The floriography, the language of
flowers, means a single red rose can communicate feelings,
the scent the ultimate scent, the rose of love can grow only
from the heart. Let the most romantic flowers on earth,
symbolize the love you share. Sprinkle rose petals on the
bed. Give your lover eleven roses and an artificial one. Tell
them you will stay in love with them until all the roses die.

Do the romantic.
Say the romantic.
Give the romantic.

Light up candles. Eat dinner by candlelight. Watch romantic

movies, for an entire day. Bring home an unexpected present. Go out on a date in the middle of the week. Do something spontaneous like giving them a big public kiss. Hold hands. Write "I love you" on the bathroom mirror. Leave a note on the car windscreen. Romantic elements add a sensual dimension to difficult times. Make a move. Do something sensual together. That's essential.

Chocolate

Do the romantic.

Say the romantic.

Give the romantic.

Tweet Tweet

Screen-time over quality time. Let's face it. You can't communicate when you are checking the iPhone or while you're on Safari online shopping. If every relationship problem starts with poor communication, you have to pay more attention to each other than your electronics. Iphones don't have feelings. If you or your partner is addicted to cyberspace, the satisfaction of receiving messages or reading posts from friends, this might be replacing the excitement between you. It looks like you're more interested in what's happening on Facebook than looking into the face of your partner. Set up some rules to stop devices getting in the way of love. Close the laptop and open up sexy two-way communication, unplug the TV; turn each other on instead.

Tweet Tweet

iPhones don't have feelings.

Cyberspace creates space between you.

Chunky Love

Are you constantly telling each other...

"That's it.
Farrrk you!
We're finished.
It's over.
Forget it."

If these are your terms of endearment...

Whatever!

What's the point of investing emotional time, if love isn't going anywhere? You can be in love one moment. Out of love the next. In love. Out of love. In. Out. The reality is, you're having a series of short-term relationships within the same tenuous relationship. Relationship status should be a given. Not up for manipulation or worries.

Emotional continuity is vital for a long term relationship, otherwise, you'll constantly worry, the worst case scenario will happen… your partner walks out of your life and slams the door. So stop unlocking the rush of negative thinking that when the going gets tough, someone will call it quits. Stop playing with the idea of leaving. Make the decision to definitely go, or definitely stay. But definitely, don't make threats. Someone might take you up on it!

Instead, do the opposite. Be a lover, not a leaver. Promise to never threaten the other with walking out the door sometime in the future. This promise of stability, by its very nature, knowing that you will love each other tomorrow, has a miraculous way of recreating an ongoing love bond. Make a pact to stay together knowing you can work through anything. A commitment to stay *twogether* is one of the most significant things you can do to create true longevity for your relationship.

Chunky Love

Be emotionally reliable.

Never threaten to quit.

Be a lover not a leaver.

Lip Attack

OK, so you share your most personal thoughts with your partner. And what happens? Inside this intimate setting, your partner does an 180° attitude change towards you; a criticism, a snappy answer will do it; it can happen anytime; feelings become confused; nasty stuff is said.

One partner may provoke an argument and then refuse to discuss the issue further. This is the partner you can't stand. Or understand. Instead of ignoring their hissy fit, you can't help yourself. You're waiting for the opportunity to step into their place of tension ... you love and hate it. You retaliate ....now there's open hostility.

Sometimes, we often create problems that don't exist or exaggerate problems that are already there. We turn stepping stones into stumbling blocks, just because we feel like it. Arguments separate you from each other. What you believe is the uniqueness of your love, is now questionable.

When you argue you must take care. What is said is never forgotten. From inside love, every word that comes out of your mouth during a heated argument is a weapon.

You say things that are false for the sting effect. Everything gets exaggerated to get a reaction. Often what is said is untrue purely to inflict emotional pain. This is the worst kind of fighting. It's unfair fighting, dirty fighting. Here the idea is not to air grievances and reach an understanding but to wound the other person as deeply as possible. This leaves too many scars. If you are not conscious of what you say, your words can hurt your partner badly. And you can't undo or unsay what you've said.

Your partner hears you loud and clear. Later you try to say:

" *I didn't really mean it...* of course it's not true!"

Too late. What's said can't be unsaid. No matter how often you say sorry, there is no easy erasure. Hurtful words turn into verbal arrows, capable of poisoning the heart. When you fire off your mouth with a grand slam attack on someone's character, you lose their trust and respect. Each time you move further away from each other and its harder to get back. So swear you'll never fire off your mouth in an argument again. It's about practicing self-control and respecting yourself and your partner.

Lip Attack

Words do kill relationships.

Once you say something, you can't unsay it.

Swear you'll never fire off your mouth again.

Inhouse Fighting

Some relationship experts tell you: to improve a relationship, simply get back to doing the little things you used to do when you first met each other. But the sad truth is, if unresolved issues keep resurfacing as arguments, no amount of favorite candy, glitterati baubles or love notes, will make any real difference. Relationships nourished solely on occasional dinners, won't cut the sugar.

Someone may think everything is fine when actually it isn't, one of you has a problem. When someone doesn't make an effort to understand your needs and feelings, it's difficult. They minimize or trivialize what you say.

If your partner avoids talking things over, you feel emotionally or verbally unheard and frustrated. You start complaining. You complain to flash a focus on what's bothering you, so they can see there is a problem. Often they still don't get the idea that anything is wrong. They are not mind readers. Many arguments are started by a partner who is frustrated with not being heard or feels they are not getting enough generous two-way talk.

You desperately want to try to overlook issues and again talk yourself out of bringing it up. But the more you hold back, the more you find yourself taking verbal swipes at your partner. Without resolution, there is a constant unnerving uncertainty. An unresolved issue never goes away on its own. It's loaded with emotional venom, ready to strike at the heart of your relationship. And with all this negative tension tightening emotional nerves, you keep waiting for someone to explode.

"You prima-donna!"
"What did you just call me...
you jerk-off?"

Arguments can get ugly and insulting. You may shout until the early hours of the morning and problems are still not resolved. In fact, your voices are set at top volume smackdown, louder than when you started.

Let's say you're passionate people and passionate people fight. Right? A shouting match is a relationship reality. We all know the initial fiery verbal outbursts and unexploded feelings burn off frustrations but deliberately shouting monologues at top voice has a tendency towards creating absolute chaos. You think shouting is the only way to let someone know how bad you feel. But while you are shouting, you can't figure out the cause of arguments, emotional intelligence is ranked zero, because the louder you shout, the less you think. That's a scientific fact. It's only when you lower your voices and both start talking again, things begin to be productive and non-threatening. It's not easy to start talking again. But talking definitely is the path to mutual understanding.

Now here's the really hard thing to do. Somewhere during the discourse of a heated argument, both apologize to each other. Say "Sorry." We are not joking! As soon as you do, you stop the ongoing collateral damage that happens when one or both holds resentment and bad feelings. Hugs also work if you can get close enough!

Neither of you should pretend what happened, didn't happen. You love each other, you can apologize to each other and it really doesn't matter who says sorry first. You're both wrong at times. The instant you both sincerely apologize, your unconditional surrender creates a new beginning. A sincere apology is an effective antidote to bad feelings and the talk becomes more intelligent, more loving.

Inhouse Fighting

Avoid being critical.

Give up the blame game.

Maintain respect for each other.

Mattress

You've heard the saying, don't go to bed without making up. Well, it's true. If you go to sleep angry, unresolved conflict goes into your psyche because our brains categorize memory, placing experiences into our long and short term memories. Sleep makes it easier to remember upsets, so if you take arguments to bed, it is more likely to get dumped into your long-term memory, where it accumulates on a deeper level; the fight holds a lasting impression and stalks your relationship from the shadows.

You can't mentally identify it, but you find yourself reacting in volatile ways towards your partner. This can happen months later and you really can't understand where these bad feelings are coming from. You'll find, not resolving differences and grievances wrecks your dreams of love. This progresses rapidly into a desire to slam the door on your intimate and physical relationship. The idea of sex goes out the bedroom window. That's why it's vital to resolve conflict on the day you argue and move past the upset. So don't ever go to bed angry, clear your negative shite before shut-eye and you won't need to count a bunch of sheep.

Mattress

Face and resolve daily issues that day.

Don't take unresolved issues to bed.

A peaceful mind makes sweet dreams.

Eat Dirt

So how do we fix things when bad feelings have
shut the relationship down to a point where you'd rather
eat dirt than saying something nice to each other! It's a
verbal fault line. A chasm as wide as it is deep. Jumping
the gap is actually quite simple. It only takes one person to
initiate discussions and close the gap between you. If you
are no good at making the first move to talk after a volatile
argument, then respect the courage it takes for your partner
to open the lines of communication. Talk about whatever
is on your mind. Conflicts get resolved by thinking and
talking honestly about what is really going on. Once you
do, you'll start sharing all your inner thoughts with renewed
truthfulness and generosity.

This disclosure of feelings moves the relationship into
deeper love and understanding. So don't be afraid to lay it all
out. Be brave! Even if your partner is saying nothing at all,
learn to read the clues. Talk it through when you are calmer
but still intense. You'll have energy and passion for doing
it. Use the energy to work it out. Use humor to resolve

conflicts. A disagreement is not about rage management. A productive fight ends in a resolution in which each person comes to understand and respect the other's point of view. When you feel truly understood and accepted, the gates to the heavenly side of your love open again. You trust each other again.

Great feelings of love return.

Eat Dirt

Say what's on your mind.

See your partner's point of view.

Jump the gap of misunderstandings.

What Would Love Do Now?

You know what a pain in the butt you can be. You
can be nasty just cause you feel like it. You can be sullen
and silent. A right shite. You may justify your response by
passing blame. Then as your partner tries to discuss things,
you take a hard tough line and become more disagreeable.
You're feeling downright tetchy: bad day at work, hard
day with the kids, your in-laws are being outlaws. Try and
remember not to shift your shite day onto your partner.
How can you expect anyone to love you when you're being
a right P.I.T.A (pain in the arse). It's easy to be a P.I.T.A.
and send bad vibes your partner's way. Every negative action
causes a negative reaction; the way an argument starts. Now
chances are you'll both end up dumping emotional trash on
each other. So many arguments stink with the compost of
unfairness to them. Whatever the reasons, remember that

you trigger each other in the positive and the negative. You know and they know, when they're being unreasonable. This is where love comes in.

When you know your partner is tired or preoccupied or just has a different opinion, be nice! Ask yourself: what would love do now? Then activate some doable thing, some loving action to reconnect. Do whatever spontaneously feels right. Let it come from the heart. You know what they like. You know when to say, let's have a hug! Make a small simple gesture. Little things count for a lot. Give some Emotional Resuscitation without hesitation. It may be as simple as a kiss!

"So how does this feel?"
"mm m mmmmmmmmmmmaaahhhhhh beautifuk."

What Would Love Do Now?

Don't dump emotional trash.

Avoid being drawn into negative vibes.

Recognize your own negativity.

Do something nice for your significant other.

Acid Rain

In unfamiliar situations, people react in different ways. Take one example of a rainy day: one person is loving the feeling of warm tropical rain on their face. Yet the other partner fears, a bolt of lightning out of the blue, is a real frightening possibility (for them).

"Really?"
"Yes really!"

Personality affects how we react to situations. Metaphorical inky dark clouds for one person is a typhoon for another. Just because you are not afraid or worried, doesn't mean you can ignore your partner's fears.

If you see your partner is stressed in a situation, don't ignore them or say...

"Don't worry, everything's OK."

Guess what? It's not OK because they're not OK. You are, but they're not. Get it? So what! Shouldn't they just get over it?

"No!"

Don't discount how your partner is feeling. Let your partner feel the fear, otherwise, you're not validating their reactions. Don't criticize your partner when they show strong emotions. If you're critical, they will see you as detached. Worse, you make them feel pathetic because they're the one voicing problems. Don't be inclined to switch off.

Let your partner be themselves. Respect your partner's uniqueness. Let them think, say and react to situations as they want to. Personal reactions never fit into neat calculations. One doesn't have to be rational, logical, or objective all the time.

Help each other out of tricky situations. We all have moments when we need to be rescued, physically, mentally or emotionally. When you give your partner support, it stops them feeling they're on their own. We all need E.R. at times. It feels good to be able to give Emotional Rescue. It's about giving a generous helping of love. Emotions are what make us human. It's safe to let feelings run as long as they aren't sweeping away the other partner in an emotional flood.

If you find yourself up against the odds, keep it real. Thinking that your partner will figure out what you need without you telling them, won't happen. When you're upset, instead of saying nothing, acting weird, freaking out and making them guess what's going on with you... tell them. Remember no one's going to read your mind! Just say one of the phrases you've agreed for situations like this:

"Acid Rain"

A saying like Acid Rain means: I need your support now, because, I'm freaking out here. It's great when a couple of words, is all you need to say to your partner...and they get where you're at immediately.

A c i d   R a i n

Be supportive.

Don't ignore your partner.

Tell your partner what's wrong.

Agree on private signals between you.

Monkey Monkey

Primitive body language is basic and can't be controlled or disguised. It's you and millions of years of human evolution. The body tells you exactly where it's at. When you sense a sensual and sexy change in body code, you can't help it, you're genetically wired to jump in. When you know someone intimately, you're acutely aware of mood changes, body language expressed through eyes, mouth, and lips; or the way someone looks at you. Good moods are so deliciously contagious, you want to share them. But it's not in your best interest to get involved with a negative mood.

Mood shifts can happen when one partner has unresolved personal issues. They can use lengthy periods of irritability, aloofness, withdrawal and negativity to bring you down. Often the mood is blamed on you, you'll struggle to understand what you did because likely you didn't do anything to set them off. It's a natural reaction to cater to the mood maker, but avoid taking any blame because moodiness thrives on exactly that.

Don't jump in if your partner is in a negative mood because unfortunately, it can be contagious. Contagious like the flu. If you catch a bad mood then you're both down with it. You're not an M.D are you? A Mood Doctor. It's not up to you to change someone's negative mood. It's up to them to sort out their own stuff. Give a person space. They'll sort it out, without you!

So what about those who love alternating between warmth and coldness, languishing in long moods. You never know that mood is next. Long moody episodes create emotional pollution that sends contradictory and confusing messages. Unvoiced negative moods get heavy and dark. They create an invisible disturbance around the place. One partner is left guessing why the other is acting like this. And no matter how hard they try to shake the happy rattle, the moody one is unsmiling. Which leaves the other one wondering, why? Are they mad at me?

"What did I do?"

You rewind the days conversations in your mind just trying to figure out the cause of prevailing moodiness.

Some partners are masters of the long sulk. They make a conscious decision to use a long moody sulk to force an issue. These moods can be weapons to get what they want. This can be as material as pressuring someone to be more agreeable to the latest mobile phone or as physical as sex or emotional as wanting more attention. They withdraw into monosyllables and turn the relationship into a strategy game.

It's all so tedious and they know it! That's the point.

You've heard that expression, "She's such a moody person." "He's always packing a sad." Constant moodiness starts to look like your personality trait. It shows and everyone can see it. No one can satisfy you. You become known as a person with a personality problem. Eventually, your partner loses respect and closes off emotionally and physically because you are too difficult to live with.

Partners want more jazz in their life. That's why constant moody blues sessions erode the intimate bond necessary for a long term loving relationship. If you're in a regular bad mood, take note. Instead of spending time sulking, why not just say…

"This bothers me… and here's why…"
"I'd like this to happen… and here's why!"

Accept the fact that you do need to discuss what's going on with you. Then instead of playing moody blues alone, you can play with each other.

Monkey Monkey

Give each other space.

Talk about how you're feeling.

Don't use moods as a weapon.

Wall Of Silence

You: "That's a great looking island!"
Partner: (No response)
You: "It'd be a great place to go
for a vacation... don't you think?"
Partner: (Silence)
You: "Well, what do you think of my
butt?"
Partner: (No response)

If you don't bother to talk, you become the silent wall. You make your partner feel like a bore; it can turn a normally calm and self-assured partner into a person who feels a neediness. They end up running monolog after monolog because you don't respond. If you reply from behind a book; don't look up from your laptop; walk into another room while they're talking; or disappear to the corner store only to return two hours later, you're guilty of giving them the silent treatment.

If you ignore your partner like this: show lack of interest, limit affection, ration out compliments or show a lack of desire for closeness you're building a great wall between you. Bigger than the wall of Mexico. It's difficult for anyone to be close and intimate when they are up against an avoidant and disinterested human wall making it impossible to scale. Through silence or nonparticipation, even if you're saying nothing, you are saying a hell of a lot. When you doodle, look at your watch or file your nails, body language says you're half listening or not listening at all. Your partner interprets your vacant sign as this. What you're doing is more important than what they have to say.

Wrong!
Wrong!
Wrong!

And when they get upset, you tell them to calm down! What causes the problem here? Silence is a distancing style of behavior. This creates emotional stress. What's more, if you don't listen with interest, it seems like your partner is not important enough to hear. The inability to listen to your partner create a poignant loss. You don't realize how damaging this vacuum is to the essential dynamics of a relationship. In the end, neither of you can talk to each other anymore. You forget how to relate because you forgot to talk. If you quit talking, you lose the person you are in love with. Communication is an art form. Express yourself and stay open to the self-expressions of others.

Wall Of Silence

Be generous in conversations.

A good listener makes a great lover.

Use small talk to bring you together.

Communication is an art form.

Knife Point

Do you find, when your partner asks you a question, they cut in with their own answer to their own question?

"Excuse me! Why ask me in the first place?"

Or interjects in the middle of a sentence before you finish what you are saying. They cut you off without a thought.

Interruptions are rude for starters; uncaring and uninvolving. By not giving someone a chance to answer, it indicates that one partner's response is not worth hearing or even considering. This may seem a small point, but the point is, devilish things are in the smallest details.

Cutting someone off is a serious disconnection because you're cutting them out. When you ask a question, wait a moment. Be interested enough to hear what your partner has to say. It's possibly sharper than you think.

Knife Point

Practice listening more and interrupting less.

Don't cut your partner off.

Dirty Flirting

Are you wondering what it would be like to be with someone else? Is the bush greener on the other side. Is the seven-year itch real? Do you secretly wonder if this has been a mistake? What if this person isn't the one? Is there someone else? Are you supposed to be with someone else?

"Shite!"

Am I wasting my life by staying? Thinking that you have made the wrong decision can keep you from appreciating the relationship you're in. You stay alert and on the lookout. You make serious eye contact with someone else and before you know it…you're dirty flirting, with all its sex, lies and compromise.

Real love turns into a mirage when you think about being someone else. You kill beautiful feelings every time you do it. When energy for your existing relationship drains away on fantasies, your feelings towards your partner and their feelings towards you get seriously diluted.

So think about long term consequences before you think about having sex with every woman man woman who looks your way. And when you are caught out, it's not good enough to say:

"Ah come on! You're imagining it!"

Flirting blurs the edges of your relationship. It affects the feelings between you both before you realize it. You can't even be imaginatively unfaithful and think you'll get away with it. Flirting embeds itself between you, damaging trust and intimacy.

Suspicion creates an invisible line between you. You know nothing is going to happen, but your partner doesn't. There may be nothing wrong with hanging out with a friend of the opposite sex. However, you need to pay attention to how even the legitimate and seemingly innocent things you do affect your partner. It's the feeling you dismiss as irrational, that create distance between you.

commitment is 90% of love

If you are a cheater in the relationship: one-night stands, internet relationships including sexting, long and short term affairs, you have to stop and leave the affair behind. If you're not committed in body, heart, and mind, then you block long-term love. There's no getting around that one. It's an absolute no-no. So stop with the flirting, cheating and imagining! Love the one you're with.

Dirty Flirting

If you're flirting...then you're hurting.

Don't screw up your relationship.

Love the one you're with.

Amnesia

Does your partner appear to have selective amnesia? You tell them something important and a few days later they say, "You never told me that!" It seems they only heard what they wanted to and didn't remember most of what you said. In this type of communication breakdown, one partner is often the parrot, regularly repeating themselves in order to be understood. You can live with someone, but not really share a full life, because of problems with all important two-way communication.

Just because you are with someone, doesn't mean to say you are in touch with each other. Two people can be together in the same house and be living emotionally alone within the relationship. It happens to be true!

Anyone can be lonely in love.

The loneliness comes from knowing you can't contact another person's feelings, no matter how hard you try. Not being able to really talk about deeper thoughts and feelings, makes for a lonely time.

Keep in mind, physical and emotional bonds are nurtured through attentive, effective communication. Communication is the glue that bonds your relationship together. Without this kind of foreplay, things get really screwed up. Make space to communicate. Take time out over coffee, put down the magazine, mute the remote. Really listening to each other, deepens the love between you.

Amnesia

Get communicating.

Be attentive and learn to listen.

Free Riding

"I want love."

"Sure thing. Of course."

"I want money."

"Yeah, yeah."

"I want a new car."

"Yeah, yeah."

"I want you to make me happy."

"Yeah, yeah."

"I want good times."

"Yeah, yeah."

Are you the partner constantly making demands? If you are, you're in a one-way relationship. All your way! Ask yourself... are you a hot or cold person in this relationship? Warm people respond to others. Cold people never act out of spontaneity but out of an instinct for self-preservation or ultimate gains. When you have a self-serving agenda, it's impossible to keep a relationship intimate and personal. When you are acquisitive, you accumulate things, not love. You're a taker, not a giver.

Is this you?

Or your partner? Lack of responsibility from one partner regarding finances and money issues, has the princess or prince attitude, all about me, all glittering and paparazzi. Making sure all wants and desires are met is just an unending list: vacations, clothing, cars, bills, household expenses, mortgages, savings, investments, money. But sooner or later, the partner's ability to service constant demands wears out, their resources, like themselves, get used up and exhausted. They wake up and look at themselves in the mirror. And then take a long hard look at the situation. They resent the lack of support. They're convinced this is not love, as they turn away.

If you want love to outshine the Lamborghini, dump the I want, more and more attitude. Get real! Life can be tough enough without you adding to it. Don't expect your partner to do all the work and all the providing. A balanced relationship is one with two equal contributors. That's the way to create a rich and fulfilling life together.

Free Riding

Keep it real.

Don't be a freeloader.

Share responsibilities.

The Leader

All intimate relationships are about power. Power shared. Power taken. Power given away. In the context of a relationship conversations and body language between you, makes the dialogue of power. Both partners need to have equal decision-making power, but often one person in the relationship dominates; by being more determined; by using a stronger more distinctive voice; by having the first and last say. Having to negotiate every situation with a power play partner is exhausting. It makes life difficult. However, if one person is dominating, they may be equating intimacy with a form of license to be the leader. In this case, there may as well be only one person in the relationship. The Leader. It's all about them.

"But what if I am the leader... gotta problem with that?"

"Well yeees!"

Is your pure brilliance the right way to do things? Not necessarily. The leader always thinks they have a faster, better answer to all situations and takes on the responsibility to ensure their brilliant idea is followed through. The know it all attitude, acting arrogant, negating, or looking for a way to one-up whatever a partner says, can become a drudge of a habit to be around. This is not what should happen in a shared relationship. If this is going on, you'll have one thing going for you.

My big fat resentment.

The Leader all power and controlling. The partner all emotional withholding. Both are power plays. There are no winners. No one should be the supreme boss of the household or for that matter, boss of someone else. No one should cultivate or maintain a power play attitude. You both walk the planet in your own way and you're both brilliant. There are no bosses here; only lovers who need to share ideas and decide things together.

The Leader
Equality rules.

See Red

"SEE!"

Look what you've made me do now!

The metaphor of the back seat driver scenario (yes, we all do it) is a huge cause of public arguments and embarrassing flare-ups, manifesting crazy dramatic outcomes for ordinary moments. Like quietly parking the car on the parallel or ramming the red battle wagon into the municipal parking meter on purpose. Then you drag the steaming battle home, like pugilistic takeaways, to fight over it for hours. Dramas make doing things together tense and less fun. Embarrassing each other with a public scene is a power play. Pretty soon you start making excuses to leave one or other at home.

You know when the metaphoric back seat driver is back, right on your back, you hear them right behind you, yacking away. They've got answers to questions you didn't even ask, telling you what to do and how to do it. And isn't it amazing…when you are on your own how you manage to be in control, stay in control and survive, without those helpful suggestions!

The way you do something is often totally different to how someone else does it. We're not clones and we're not robots. Everybody does things differently. Butt out. Resist looking over your partner's collarbone and vice versa.

Interfering while someone is trying to negotiate tricky situations, creates confusion and frustration. The partner who is trying to sort things out doesn't need quips, interjections, or smart answers from you. So if you try and help someone when they haven't asked, you signal a lack of belief in them. What can you do when someone's interfering, while you are doing, what you do?

You just gotta say...

"Who's in the driver's seat? Me!
Who's in the back seat? You!
Hands off the controls."

It goes like this: when someone is in control, let them drive the car, find a car park, book the hotel, choose the wine and complain about the food. Let the starter finish whatever they are doing without receiving the verbal assistance they never actually asked for. Give them the respect and space to do things their way.

See Red

Don't tell your partner what to do or how to do it.

Let your partner finish what they've started.

The Cereal Talker

"Blah Blah Blah Blah Blah Blah Blah Blah Blah Blah Blah Blah Blah Blah Blah Blah Blah Blah Blah"

If you do all the talking what's up? If you are telling your partner how it is from the minute they wake up; over espresso, over toast, over eggs, over and over, till the light goes out, then sure as eggs, you're the one more interested in doing the talking than listening. Some people give no respite from the blah blah; once on a verbal roll, they choose to announce every little thing they are thinking and what's more, talk about everything they're going to do or not do. When their news is switched on all day; you switch off.

Right?

Listening to continual information makes it difficult to differentiate verbal chatter from the need to engage in important discussions. A busy mind filled with monkey chatter leaves no space for exchanging meaningful ideas and thoughts. Instead of constantly talking at your partner and expecting them to fulfill all your needs for personal expression, allow each other space and time out. No matter how much you want to be with someone, take the time to relax. Look after yourself. When you have balance and equilibrium in your own life, you bring meaningful expression into your relationship.

Talking about meaningful dialogue, keep the *blah blah blah* out of your bedroom too. Talk body language only.

The Cereal Talker

Give each other time out.

Make your bed a blah blah free zone.

Give each other verbal relief.

Emotional Library

In every relationship you've ever had, including this one, you have experiences which you retain as memory. All of these personal experiences are stored in the vault of yourself. Some people call it emotional baggage. We prefer to call it the emotional library; where every experience, every reflection, every argument, every joke is filed away as a memory. The problem happens when you come face to face with a difficult situation, it's all too easy to pull down a volume of experiences from another relationship and cross-reference it to the one you're in.

How easy is it to overlay your previous responses onto situations now. Way too easy and it's so wrong. When you filter everything through your catalog of past experiences, you're not connecting up in a fresh new way as a couple. New experiences challenge us every day, which means we are constantly developing and changing as people. And we need to embrace this. Change renews us. In fact, every seven years our bones, muscles, and tissues renew themselves. So does our heart. Change is also part of moving on in any relationship. Part of moving on is about leaving things behind, especially previous lovers. Yet, some people inadvertently or blatantly invite their past lovers back into their current relationship, by talking them up or down to the new lover. Often they use social symbols to do it. How strong, how sexy, how rich, how handsome, how beautiful, how talented, how adventurous, they all were.

If you have a habit of talking about your previous partners, what are you really doing? Are you subconsciously trying to shape your present partner into the best of your past lovers? Is this what you want? How does your present partner feel about that? Make a decision to shelve previous relationships. The relationship script is being written all the time. See your partner as they are right now. Don't use the out-of-date defunct stuff. Use the new and funky. This makes room for a whole new love story.

Emotional Library

See your partner as they are right now.

Don't overlay past relationships on this one.

Make a decision to shelve past relationships.

WeWe

When you met, you were attracted to the fascinating person who was living their own life. Then We jumped into bed. We were so into each other. We began to blend ourselves into one homogeneous couple.

We think

We eat

We go

We drink

We have

We drive

We do

We like

We're not individuals.

We're WeWe!

"WeWe?"

"Yes. What?"

"How did this happen WeWe?"

"Because we love each other! Don't we WeWe?"

Then WeWe decided those unusual charming character traits must go.

"Like that crazy laugh of yours. That turkey laugh is not allowed out of the house."

"Well, then neither are those yellow flip-flops you bought on sale!"

Yes. WeWe needed to change things around here. Like you! And you! This pattern of trying to change each other for the better is one of the worst things you can do in a relationship. You simply forget who you are in relation to each other. Nothing about your identity should have to change dramatically because you are together. A relationship can grow and develop far beyond ordinary possibilities. To make this happen, you need to do two things.

First, be yourself by getting rid of WeWe. Make a point of maintaining your own quirky habits. Stay weird if that's what you like. The way you do things is unique and part of your identity. A sense of yourself gives you self-esteem. A full quota of self-esteem is empowering. You drive your own destiny and encompass others in your future plans, including your lover. When two lovers realize their full potential as individuals, your partnership has double the strength. It gives you power *twogether* to adapt to any social physical or emotional dynamics in life. As strong individuals, you make a formidable team, ready for any challenges. Whether it's a new baby, a new job, or winning the lottery.

Second, open your eyes and take a closer look at the special individual you fell in love with. Celebrate your differences; outlooks, interests, beliefs, the things that attracted you to each other in the first place.

WeWe

Keep your own quirky habits.

Be more of who you are not less of yourself.

If you must change someone, look in the mirror.

Space

Time apart is important in a relationship, your free time is your free time. Having interests outside the relationship is like coming up for air. When a partner doesn't want you out of their sight to allow you to do something on your own it can create an issue. Sacrificing your own need for space, to keep the peace, is not an answer. One partner has to give up fears about the other doing things on their own. Building trust between you is the answer.

Taking time out doesn't mean where you go and what you do should be a great mystery. The difference between privacy and secrecy is this. A relationship is about sharing and openness. Secrecy can leave your partner feeling emotionally abandoned. Keep and develop trust with each other by doing what you say. Be consistent. Be on time. Do what you say you will. Call when you say you will. Take time to remember who loves you! Love and trust between you are built up this way.

Spend time apart, but not so much that you drift apart. Take time out and share time together.

Space

Stay in touch.

Build trust.

Be reliable.

Don't be secretive.

P.K.

Do you like spontaneity? Like bumping into a best friend you haven't seen since high-school, on the third floor of the MoMA Gallery, at three thirty-five on a Thursday afternoon, looking at a Matisse. What are the odds of that?

weirdcrazyconnections

are what we call P.K. moments.

Those personal Pre-disposed Kinetic times when the earth seems to rotate on its axis, just for you. Those moments born from a gut feeling to do something, like phoning a friend you suddenly think about. And as soon as they speak, you know in a nanu the reason you had to call. But, how hard is it to act on spontaneous feelings, when you have a partner who's always making, yet another helpful, useful, thoughtful, better suggestion. By interfering with your plans and suggesting alternatives, which may inadvertently stop you making the P.K. connection. If you don't follow your gut feeling, that split second in time, just for you, vanishes. The syncronistic nature of your own life doesn't have a chance to happen.

Rare moments are rare and can easily be get missed in a moment. P.K. is the freedom to respond to your intuition. That way you can master your own universe and share the surprising experience you've had when you come back.

P . K .

Respond to intuition.

Let spontaneity into your life.

Allow your partner to follow their intuition.

Rubber
Glove

As two individuals, you have different abilities, likes, and dislikes. You do what you do best. You take domestic roles by informal mutual agreement. You live together. It's part of the deal. At some point, you both agreed, that one person can do some things better than the other. Which was fine. Power was still relatively equal. You understood job allocations, it made perfect sense, household responsibilities equally distributed. But wait a moment:

"Why have I still got the rubbish job?"

At first, driving the big white porcelain bus...i.e cleaning the toilet was OK but scrubbing the loo three times a week adds up to one hundred and sixty-two times a year of toilet brushing! Now that's just shitty.

Sure things have to be done, but how about swapping jobs around. You clean the bathroom; I'll put the trash out; you wash the car; I'll wash the dog; you barbecue; I'll pick up the laundry; you get the idea. Swap household duties about. When the yellow rubber glove's on the other hand, you gain an instant appreciation for what each person contributes to the practical side of your relationship. In a few weeks, you'll notice the energy levels in the relationship improve 100% when you clear the air and refresh the dusty musty things.

We're adding one more scenario into the domestic scene: One person's decided it's time to vacuum the living room. You're sitting relaxing with your feet up. You can see them from your place on the sofa. Very sucky-moto, heading your way (just to make you feel bad). Tension and intention rise as you lift your feet. It's not how they do it, it's the attitude they bring with the *suck-shin...fuuu*k!* You can avoid the cleaning guilt trip when you both agree to:

Do it with love or don't do it at all!

So when you see one person dragging the vacuum cleaner like a dog on a rope, don't feel guilty or afraid they're on your case. Remember they're doing it with love, so relax.

One person is not pretending... they love to do it!

Now all you lazy shites are thinking... great! One person loves to do it, so, one person can do it all the time. Wrong. Un-velcro your ass from the sofa. No slackers! Doing it with love is only for people who love their home and harmony.

Rubber Glove

Exchange responsibilities.

Do it with love or don't do it at all.

Lipstick

"Does this look good on me? does my hair look OK? are my undies showing through? is there lipstick on my teeth?"

Wait a minute. If you invite your partner to keep an eye on your physical appearance, they'll develop a seriously bad habit of constantly checking you out. They'll be in your face 24/7 because you gave them permission to be your personal groomer. If you slide under their microscope, you're under observation. You've created a situation. Sometimes you want to kick back and relax and have a bad hair day. But if you've put someone on high alert, they think you want to look great all the time. Allow them to be your body critic and before you know it, they'll upscale comments to:

"You're looking a bit porky... just thought you should know."
!!!!!!!!???

Don't ask your partner to be your talking mirror. Your partner is not trained to be your make-over artist, oral hygienist, dresser or makeup artist. Or for that matter, your private mime artist; running their tongue over their ivories in an effort to show, *you've got one black cumin seed caught between your teeth… just thought you should know!*

There have been great mime artists in the world and your partner isn't one of them. So stop asking your partner to be your minder. Or they'll end up being your body critic.

Lipstick

Look out for yourself.

Stop making your partner your body critic.

Zig Zag

When you met you were total strangers. Now you can see the outline of each other's smile with your eyes closed. When you know someone intimately, you're in sync. You seem to know what the other is going to say before they've said it. You find yourselves finishing each other's sentences, at times it's perfectly seamless as if you've got the same heartbeat. It's a beautiful thing. Then one partner starts to think their way is better. They begin to re-vamp your ideas.

"Can I ask you something?"
"Sure."
"Why is your idea better than mine?"
"Because your idea sux."
"Well... how about this, I'll never suggest anything to you again!"
"Fine. Good Idea."

SLAM

"Maybe your idea was OK after all."

Do you find when you suggest an idea, how easily someone puts forward their idea over it? No matter what you suggest, they have another suggestion. If someone always has the final say, all the decisions go one way. The oneness becomes numbness. Flatline thinking which is so disinteresting. ZZZZZZZZZZZZZZZZZZZZZZ

How boring is that? Don't discount your partner's ideas. If you don't value what your partner thinks, the mutual energy will go. You don't think or act the same as your partner. Your goals and dreams may not align exactly. That's great. You might have a wayout idea that makes your partner do a sudden double take. The voyage of the best relationship is a Zig Zag line of a hundred tacks. So why run a straight line through life. Zig Zag!

Life is incredibly interesting together. Life can be unique when you make it that way. Remember, the best relationship is a Zig Zag line of a hundred ideas and they're not all yours. A shared life is about sharing. Not shooting each other down. The idea is when someone has a plan, watch you don't smother it with alternative suggestions. If someone can be bothered to use their own brain to come up with a wonderful idea first … go with it. Try not to adapt, change, or alter them. This means, if it's Goan chicken curry at Little India, don't go on about pepperoni pizza at Ginos. Make the first idea put forward on the table, the one you agree with. And next time, when you suggest a flight of fancy first, they'll happily go along with you.

Something to note about putting forward singular ideas as a couple. It's not what you say, it's how you say it. When you have a thought, don't present it as a question. It's like putting forward an idea and asking someone to judge it. Should we? Can we? Do you think? How about? What do you think? Forget these continuous ????????????????????????? ?????????????????? It's so tempting, you can expect to have your idea critiqued and possibly have your mind changed. To stop someone changing the idea you came up with, be more up front. Make a definite point of saying what it is you want.

Zig Zag

Love is a journey. Not a destination.

Zig Zag two ways: Your way and their way.

Peaches
& Pears

What has a can of peaches got to do with you guys? Or a can of plums or pears, or apricots. More than you think! In the Garden of Eden, lovers are talking ad infinitum about a whole basket of consumer items in the local supermarket.

"Do you prefer curly or straightening shampoo?"

"What! I'm follically challenged!"

"Peppermint or whitening toothpaste or the one with fresh breath stripes."

"No, I'm bored with that."

"What kind of toilet paper do you want Seashells? Stars?"

"You pay for patterns.
"How about embossed white?"
"Boring."
"What about recycled? Shite head!"

What say you stop making mutual decisions about domestic nothings. It doesn't take two massive human brains to make these decisions. It's not domestic physics. It's supermarket shopping!

There's nothing sadder than seeing two intelligent people talking about toilet paper at great lengths! It gets worse. Check out couples doing shopping, one pushing the trolley, one pointing blankly at cans on shelves, trying to get to one mutual mind numbing minor decision over pears, plums, apples, apricots, peaches or pink guavas.

"Syrup?"
"Juice."
"Sliced?"
"Whole."
"Organic?"
"If you say so."

Claustrophobic thinking happens when you both do something that doesn't need *twogetherness,* en meme temps *(of the same breath).* You don't need a mutual agreement to buy toothpaste or a cake of soap. Why not have different kinds of toothpastes, two handmade soaps on a rope and keep nourishing the honeyed art of making personal choices. Not every carton of milk needs to be homogenous. Shopping is just one example of how you can keep both keep your individual tastes and preferences happening. You don't have to agree on everything as a couple. Why not take turns bringing home the bacon, take turns stopping off at the deli on your way home from work, or shop online and take delivery.

When you do happen to pass through the doors of the supermarket together, take a shopping cart each and start at two different food locations. One starts in the fruit department. The other begins with a loaf at the bakery. You'll be surprised at how little of these you double-up on.

You'll discover you don't actually have to be side by side to make joint decisions on the small print. You'll also find out what your partner loves and hates; their secret passion for banana custard, baby food, blue corn taco chips, black jelly-beans and green jelly babies. You'll learn more about who they truly are and they'll know your penchant for Beluga caviar on black rye with a shot of Russian Vodka.

There is only one rule when you shop; your partner must accept what you buy and vice versa.

Peaches & Pears

Make individual choices.

Your partner has personal obsessions. So do you.

Eat. Love. Enjoy.

The Sleeper

Yawn
Yawn
Yawn
(lazy partners)

They often ask questions like … What's for dinner?
How does this work? Can you fix this? One partner becomes
the sleeper. The other becomes...the expert. Like a specialist
in the relationship, the expert is always asked about specific
things. They become the maitre de, the epicurean authority,
the horticulturists with the green thumb, the mechanic
and tire repair specialist. One partner relies on the other's
expertise. While it sounds practical, we believe it turns the
relationship into a sleepy backwater.

Now imagine having two individuals in the relationship who both know how things work. You both understand widgets, organic composting. Four green hands instead of one green thumb. Your ordinary kitchen becomes a souped-up kitchen with two great chefs stirring and sautéing different dishes. Now you have a much more dynamic scenario.

Do research; gain knowledge and make decisions. Use your own creative juices. Share your ideas. Stimulating the senses makes you more intelligent. Even if you don't notice a change in I.Q. quota, you'll definitely have a great time admiring each others bonsai and eating each other's goulash.

The Sleeper

Extend your abilities.

Break out creative juices.

Make individual decisions.

Stimulate your relationship I.Q.

Are You OK?

Treat each other like the best friends you are. Friends are genuinely interested in how you feel. They try hard to find out what is inside. Friends take turns talking and listening. When you speak up and express opinions, friends don't get uncomfortable, they get interested, they make a point of getting involved in the subject, whatever the topic. So pick up on the subjects your partner initiates. Break the habit of greeting a comment with silence. Take what they say seriously. And show it by being interested. It works both ways. Share the past and present experiences and dreams for the future. When you get to talking in a relaxed open way like you do with a best friend, eighty-two percent of your relationship problems will be solved (or there about). What can you do right now to improve your relationship?

It's really simple. Ask the question...

"So...how are you doing?"

It says I'm interested and I care about you.

Are You OK?

Listen and speak the way a friend does.

Get interested and get involved.

Love In

Without sharing an intimate life, a couple can become disconnected to the point where they're just not into each other anymore. Then little by little, you stop sharing most things in your relationship. You become so distant you can't see what you are as a couple anymore.

Three lovebuster alerts you need to be aware of!

First, you let your sex life slip below the radar. You don't need each other as much as you used too. Then, you adjust to the lack of interest and lose interest. Finally, you find it impossible to recover what you have with your partner. Next thing you know, you're splitting up.

Sure, you get busy. Your partner makes adjustments when you're working all hours. They start accepting without complaint when you say you are too tired to make love. They stop complaining and telling you they want to spend more time with you. They give up expecting you to be there for them. Eventually, it occurs to you to put more effort into the relationship. You plan to take a week off only to find out that your partner has made other plans. They no longer wait till you switch off the computer, turn off the TV and feel in the mood. They adapt to the fact that you are only there, sometimes, physically or emotionally for them. But not enough to make them feel desired and sexually fulfilled as a lover. The sad part is, they adjust their emotional needs to not needing you. You both start feeling out of touch and in the worst case scenario, estranged from each other. You end up doing more things separately and you can end up so apart as a couple, that you end up separating and going different ways. When you take your sexual connection for granted, you can lose what you have.

Do it or lose it!

Sex shouldn't be the last thing you do before falling asleep. The last thing you think of as you turn off the light. Often one partner complains that they are too tired to make love. And the other person has a headache. So days turn into weeks and weeks into months and before you know you are making love once a month. Life gets in the way of lovemaking. Yet, sex is critical to a great, long-lasting relationship. Neglect sex and everything eventually supersedes sex. Until one day you realize that you haven't made love for two weeks, two months, two years or longer. Notice how grumpy you both get when you don't have sex. How fights develop out of the blue often because you want to get close, but you're both untouchable!

No loving couple can afford to neglect the sex. This is the basic secret to an intimate sexual relationship. No matter how much money you make, and the effort, energy and time it takes to make it, there is an essential rule in life here. You can't buy what a great sex life gives you. It is so valuable, that to neglect your sex life, or think it isn't as important as your workout in the gym or playing eighteen holes on the golf course is erroneous, which of course is the complete opposite of erogenous! Neglecting the bedroom is one of the biggest mistakes you can make. Sex benefits your relationship, both in and out of the bedroom. Starve each other of a physical relationship and you'll feel empty of love.

When this happens, it's not the end. You need to up your sex quota. Make love more and you will feel more in love. Get back in touch. Having a store of erotic feelings gained from making love, helps you cope with the not-so-great parts of your life. Spend more intimate hours in the soft warmth of each other's arms. Put sex in your day. Notice how small stuff, ego issues, seem to matter less.

Love is a banquet.
Indulge

Don't go hungry or run on empty. The idea is to do the opposite.

Value your sexual relationship above all else. Make time for making love. Don't let too much time pass between you without making a sexual connection. Keep kissing. Kissing is an exchange of hormones that heightens your sexual drive and focus. Keep sex a current topic. Talk about sex for 5 minutes every day. Read up on sex. It is well documented that a passionate, intimate, healthy sex life is the key to long-term relationships. You feel loved and feelings of love are felt and returned by your partner.

Love In

Great intimacy creates great passion.

Great love is within you both.

Ring A Bell?

Are your fights getting dirty and hitting below the belt?

Make an effort to keep all your fights clean. Don't disrespect the person you love. If you verbally or emotionally attack when you argue, (instead of dealing with the issue) then you are 'Dirty Fighting.'

You say things that are false for the sting effect of getting back at your partner. You exaggerate to get a reaction. This is the worst kind of fighting. It's unfair fighting, it's dirty. If you're not conscious of what you say, your words can hurt your partner badly. This leaves the other person feeling abandoned and humiliated.

You want to be able to look back on any disagreement and not have any negative emotions. Think of words as having permanence. Chose words very thoughtfully. What you say matters. So make an effort to keep all your fights clean. Simply being aware of how you argue and setting up new ground rules is the first step in sorting out sparring matches between you.

Start by defining the problem and be as specific as you can. When two people 'define' what they want to talk about, they won't end up arguing and going over and over the same ground. Avoid general terms and your talk will become clearer and if your discussions do go off track, you won't wander far from the point. You'll go from link to link along the chain of discussion, following each others chain of thought; by the time you reach the last link in the chain, you'll understand the issue and see the point of view.

When you respect each other, you won't end up sorting out an issue through a dirty fight scene. Or worse, having a deep nagging sense that you've gained another negative perspective about your partner and your relationship. When you keep the fights clean, you forget that style or mode of retaliation. Once you set the rules and agree to make an effort to understand each other rather than create unsustainable conflict, your relationship comes out on top every time.

Argue in a way that's constructive and you intensify your interaction together. When you keep the fights clean, you and your partner fight for freedom - the freedom to deal with any problem. You solve issues with focus, simply because you avoid extended bouts of emotional conflict.

When you keep the fights clean, you'll notice how you avoid the aftermath a fight causes. Less recovery time means less time trying to make up (hours, days, weeks, months, years) and more time to make-out. Even if you haven't reached a solution and are still working on it - there is a peaceful feeling when you know your fights stay clean. No nasty verbal punches.

Ding! Ding!
No bad feelings left behind.

Ring A Bell
Keep The fights clean.

Dirty fighting breaks trust.

The
Headache

When you have the proverbial,

"Not tonight I've got a headache."

Here's the thing... sex is better than aspirin. It's the headache-free card! Having sex floods your brain with chemicals that make you feel great. You get so many great benefits: antidepressant, beautifying, longevity, anti-stress, analgesic as a bonus.

Sex is a natural drugstore, the best panacea against depression. Why? Researchers have documented a release of feel-good chemicals which dulls pain and reduces stress levels. Sex is a natural high. It elevates your mood when you're feeling down.

Life-saver sex:

Statistics show that you will live longer and stay in better shape if you are having sex. Repairs cells and renews tissues, and promotes circulation for healthy skin.

Life-guard sex:

Revives, rejuvenates. Sex can reduce the risk of stroke. Sex helps the body fight free radicals and so assists the anti-aging process. Sex boosts your immune system.

Specialist sex:

Proven to reduce the risk of breast and prostate cancer.

Doctor sex:

Helps the body heal cuts, fight infection, mend deep wounds and repair bruised tissues. Supports red and white blood cells, oxygenates blood, and promotes bone growth.

Psychologist sex:

Improves memory and cognitive skills. Sex works both ways, you feel great and your partner does too.

Personal trainer sex:

Makes you more flexible, boosts your metabolism helping you burn fat quicker and stay hardcore.

The Headache

Sex is a natural drugstore.

The Back Burner

Are you putting love on the back burner because everything else is hot to trot? How you do sex is a metaphor for how you do life.

Why is a sex life so important?

Sex is like a mirror reflecting, patterns and survival strategies seen in other areas of your life. Sex is vital to keeping your relationship *twogether.*

Making love has a cumulative effect. The more physical love you share, the greater emotional love you feel. Couples who are intimate do not put their sex life on the proverbial back-burner; they make sex the number one activity. They don't allow work and the outside world to dominate so much there's no time to get it on.

You can tell couples who have a great physical time t*wogether*. It shows because outwardly they appear more together. You can't help notice the couple who have an obvious, intimate connection between them. People often ask them, what their secret is. Easy, physical attraction, passion, intimacy and a huge helping of sex.

You feel happier, more generous, and trust yourself and others more. This happy feeling is catchy! People around you pick it up. When you're desired, wanted, loved, understood and sexually fulfilled, it shows.

Great sex is not about specific technique. Standing on your head. Swinging from the chandelier. Missionary position, lotus, warrior, down-dog up-dog. A skilled lover isn't someone who knows every position in the book, it's the lover who is fully in the moment, generous with their feelings and not holding back.

Work is work. Jobs are jobs. Money is money. Never sacrifice your love and allow work, jobs and money to replace what you have as a couple.

The Back Burner

Making love has a cumulative effect.

The more loving sex you have the more love grows.

Sexual
Allsorts

The routine of sex, while safe, can lead to sex being bottom of the list of jobs to do. Now, your once passionate encounters turn into assorted sex:

quickie sex
last minute sex
squeeze one in sex
OK sex
catch up sex
do it yourself sex
if I have to sex
if you want to sex
we haven't had sex in a while sex

Then there's the ever popular:

maintenance sex

Maintenance Sex is what couples do when they slip into a routine. Maintenance sex, is sex as most couples do it; jump into bed, turn down the light, a little foreplay, or not, kiss and get down to it. Sex happens, as soft and familiar as your favorite pillow, as comfortable as your sofa, as reliable as your grandmother's recipe for chocolate cake. Perfectly OK and pleasurable. Yeah! But can you say it's really great sex? You need to go against the idea of maintenance sex. Maintenance sex, is general upkeep sex that easily turns into once in a blue moon sex: seasonal sex; the first fall of snow, annual sex, Christmas holidays, vacation sex, birthday sex, anniversary sex. If that is all you get up too, you'll end up bored with each other.

The more you put out, the more you're going to bling in the whole sex thing. Maintain a sexual connection with your partner is all about not holding back. Maintaining a sexual connection during the day keeps a strong sense of sexuality outside of the bedroom. Foreplay serves an important purpose in the art of seduction. You trigger sex hormones that make great orgasm possible later. You can experience six times the orgasm when you practice the art of seducing each other. Latest research shows that slow, tantalizing, drawn-out foreplay releases key hormones in the brain- testosterone in a man, estrogen in a women, dopamine and oxytocin in both. When testosterone, estrogen, dopamine and oxytocin come together the result is orgasm central: explosive orgasms, simultaneous and multiple orgasms.

Sending sexy txt messages or surprising them with a sexually loaded compliment. Flirting with your partner is part of seduction. Try a sexy, direct statement, that says "I want you". Then watch the tempo go up after the usual hug and kiss. You can leave things for the imagination- whether it's whispering innuendos, or leaving a sexy note on a pillow. It doesn't take much to get someone thinking about sexy possibilities. You know what gets them excited and keeps them turned on.

Seduce and let loose!

Anything you do or say that creates erotic anticipation has the effect of foreplay on the brain. You can be apart during the day and already boosting dopamine levels that amp up your partners libido...the urges that make you want to make love. Dopamine increases, the hormone responsible for creating physical and sexual excitement. And many happy returns!

Sexual Allsorts

Money can't buy what great sex gives you.

Don't neglect sex.

Seduce and let loose!

Touch Down

Ask yourself this question: in a 24 hour day, how many times do you touch, kiss or hug each other? If the answer is... I can't remember, then remember this: no matter how long you've been together, you never outgrow your need to be in touch. Your skin is the biggest sensory organ you have, yet it's often forgotten about.

Stay in touch.

Being touched in sensual, sexual, and caring ways makes you feel relaxed, loving, and loveable. Every time you touch each other, you release a powerhouse of the hormone oxytocin- the cuddle hormone. Oxytocin makes you feel more connected to each other. The more you touch each other with skin to skin contact, the more the hormone accumulates. When you give full attention to your partner, you write your own chapters together. Intimacy, love, trust, passion and sensual liaisons give you more than physical pleasure. You find yourself sharing a deep limitless connection with your partner. This happens when both physical and emotional elements are in the right position.

Touch Down

Stay in touch.

Stay in love.

Fantasy & Ecstasy

Do you spend more time talking about work, kids, and money, than talking intimately? Sex is a relevant topic in a relationship too. Just because your sex life is fine, it doesn't mean that you should take it for granted. It's worth checking if it's in the red or the black with an intimate chat; what gives you pleasure, what feels exquisite to you, how you like to play, secrets of foreplay hidden fantasies and ecstasies.

Your relationship is your personal bank of intimate feelings. You both make withdrawals and deposits. Partners feel connected and more in tune with each other when they are free to give and say and show what they want and like. In this way, you learn how unlimited sex is.

You'll discover how you can
make love with the same lover
a thousand times and yet
the lovemaking always feels
different and new!

Fantasy & Ecstasy

Sex is a highly relevant topic.

Intimatus

You know you can be together as a couple but not intimate. Intimacy isn't just about just doing things and going places together. It's way more involved than that. When you are intimate with someone, you are literally making yourself known to your partner.

What is intimacy exactly? The word intimacy comes from the Latin intimatus. Intimatus means to make something known to someone. Intimacy begins at the start of a relationship and grows over time depending on what you put into your relationship. So the more physically and emotionally true you both are, the more intimate you are.

Intimacy is real.
You can't pretend you have it.
You can't fake it.
You've got to make it.

Every act of intimacy creates more intimacy. Each time you kiss, touch, share secrets, make love, you connect in an intimate way, you make yourself known. Get slack on intimate behavior and you are no longer contributing to deeper intimacy. So continually share the intimate. It's the way to grow a deeper feeling of love.

Intimatus

Every act of intimacy creates more intimacy more love.

Finger Print

"You piss me off!"

"You forgot to..."

"You remind me of..."

"You said..."

"You lost my..."

"You didn't remember..."

"You promised..."

"You left the..."

The most finger pointing word in the whole of the English dictionary is:

YOU!

How many times do you include the word 'you' in conversations? If the discussion turns to finger pointing, you're heading for a fight. Once you are aware of how much finger pointing, blame, and accusations belongs to the word you; you can do something about it. Make a point exactly what you mean without it sounding like an accusation.

Pointing the finger of blame is a sure way to kill any conversation about issues you wish to talk about. Don't go pointing the finger of blame at your partner, or bringing up random shortcomings that are irrelevant. Don't chip away at your partner for minor 'crimes'. Instinctively, the slightest touch of blame, moves them like a chess piece into a protective position of self-justification. You arm yourself with words, and fight back. Blame no one and your problem-solving capabilities as a couple improves dramatically. When this happens, you'll make positive changes and discover new ways to relate to each other.

Finger Print

Don't point the finger of blame.

Improve your problem-solving capabilities

Triple Trouble

Triple trouble. This is where life throws more than one problem in your direction like:

Your car breaking down, your dog running away and a serious life issue you didn't see coming!

Unforeseen and unpredictable things throw your life into complete and utter chaos. These extremely trying times test your reserves as a couple to the maximum. You can feel like two separate people, coping in your own way with life's dramas. As they unfold, you forget to look after the relationship, until eventually you no longer fall back on each other for support when you need it most. Or worse, blame each other for the situations or outcome. In times of crisis, you can start to avoid the very person who needs you and whom you need, as stress and turmoil overcome the situation. We all experience hard and difficult times throughout our lives, none of us are immune, but you can come out with your relationship still intact.

Accept that in times of crisis you'll experience strong emotions. But don't be tempted to throw any negativity in your partner's direction. If you do, you risk having a couple's breakdown on top of your current situation. Instead, make an effort to let feelings come and go. Don't act on them. Don't involve your partner until you have clarity. And when you do you'll have a friend there to discuss it with! When you suffer life dramas, it's doubly important to look after each other. Then your relationship won't be an unfortunate casualty of your circumstances.

Triple Trouble

Help each other out.

Be each other's number one supporter.

Dog With A Bone

Are you like a dog with the proverbial bone? Do you have difficulty letting go?

Do you bury things that have been said, only to dig them up later and have another go?

Do you pretend to accept apologies? Tell them you forgive them, but know you won't forget, and whenever a new argument arises, you let the ghosts of the previous discourses join in the latest argument. Then in another variation you find yourself digging up dirt from previous fight scenes and splicing them all together.

You produce the same words your partner said a few days before, or months or years, in order to contradict what they are saying. By displacing, disjointing words, and sentences, by misunderstanding the whole, or quoting only part of what was said, you may show up their inconsistencies. But you won't show them your capacity for love. When something is agreed, after a fight /discussion, post resolution of said fight, the subject should never be raised again in the same context. Know when to let go. Letting go doesn't mean you dig the parts up months later.

Just let it go.

Dog With A Bone

Don't bite the hand that loves you.

Stage Left

Shouting, name calling, slamming doors, smashing feelings, breaking trust, trashing love, throwing clothes into a bag, calling a cab for the airport; that's when a simple disagreement escalates into a dreadful scene. Fights that turn into dramas, build up in your mind. It's not good. The more crap, the more negative dossiers, and scripts accumulate and collect in your memory, the dramas receive no critical acclaim for love. They spotlight the worst of you. One scene follows another until your relationship is like a sad B grade movie. A bad, ugly, embarrassing one you've produced. Dramas are the sticks and stones that damage love. If you could take photographs of the dramas, they would make a big black yearbook of bad feelings. Accumulating bad feelings is not the aim of a long-term loving relationship. Arguments that attack on a personal level are destructive enough to destroy love. In that case, there are no oscar winners. You both lose big time.

Every emotional scene you make is distressing and every scene you participate in has the potential to end the relationship. You never know which drama will be the deciding factor for your partner. The point when they have had enough of you! An emotional tipping point where you can't go back to how things were. Every uncensored argument breaks down good feelings between you. Too many dramas and couples are ready to sign each other out of their lives.

Intelligent loving means you roadblock any arguments before they turn into a drama. If you can't let things go, make sure you prevent them escalating into major dramas. You have it in your power to stop the high drama.

Apply the 30 - minute rule.

After 30 minutes, when disagreements are going nowhere;

STOP.

Take some physical time-out from each other. Agree to talk about it in 1 hours time. Get back together. Talk for 30 minutes. If you still haven't figured it out leave it. Arrange an exact time and perhaps another day to talk about the issue. After 30-minutes, apply the 30-minute rule again.

Stage Left

Emotional scenes are love wreckers.

Don't let arguments turn into dramas.

Apply the 30-minute rule.

Five Sides

Arguments don't start by themselves. We make them happen. Before you know, it's a rabble-rousing domestic relentless incendiary involving:

The Perpetrator
The Victim
The Avenger
The Rescuer
And Victim #2!

There are five sides to every argument because most arguments go like this: The Perpetrator is upset or outraged about something. They might have held their feelings inside but now reach their flash point where they say something outrageous and provocative to the victim.

The Victim (who may have their feet up reading a book and relaxing) is immediately turned into: The Avenger.

The Avenger's automatic reaction is to get pay-back. When this happens, The Perpetrator, (remember the one who brought up the issue in the first place) seeing the anger they have caused, starts to feel guilty. The Perpetrator quickly becomes The Rescuer.

The Rescuer feels bad about what is happening, and at the same time, frustrated because they still haven't sorted the problem they brought up in the first place. The whole situation gets messy. They still have a problem and they've turned their targeted victim into an aggressor. The solution for The Rescuer at that point is to take the role of The Victim to calm The Aggressor down, with not a solution in sight. How insane is that!

A Couple's argument has four sides. In any disagreement, you can identify The Perpetrator, The Avenger, The Rescuer and The Victim. Go figure. Now Pandora's Box of arguments is laid out flat, you can both step outside the square and find answers to the meaningless mess.

Five Sides

Don't box yourselves into an argument.

One Sentence

As a couple, you experience good times and bad. When you talk about the good times together, those thoughts trigger feel-good chemicals. But, if you talk about the stressful times, like the time when you lost your job, or when your business went under, or the family crisis, by the time you finish talking over the past, it creates a cocktail of stress chemicals in your body. You will feel as stressed out as when the event took place. You feel miserable again.

Talking about the bad, the difficult and the stressful times can become a habit. But giving up this addiction to unresolvable stressors, is actually easier than you think. First become aware of the stressful topics you drag up and chew over a lot, the ruminating ones: lawyer, boss, business, friends, money, ex-lover, bills, or the interferring mother-in-law. Be aware that certain trigger words lead on to extended stressful conversations. Then, when you happen to be talking and recognize a key trigger word, you can say:

"One Sentence."

Which means saying one sentence only about the stressful topic. That sentence only... about mom!. That's absolutely it for the trigger topic. And neither of you pursue the topic at that point in time. Later, of course, but not now.

This stops the ruminating in endless discussions over past events that you can't change, no matter how many times you bring them up and go over them. Some things just make you feel sad and bad. Don't allow stressors to sneak back into your conversation.

If you want to discuss a key trigger topic, ask permission from your partner to talk about an issue, so they can be mentally prepared and emotionally ready to discuss it. Find a place outside the house to talk over negative stressful issues. Keep your house for positive times, then you won't end up filling your living environment with negativity. Bad feelings and memories accumulate like static in a house. It's the number one reason why most people move house or their relationships without ever knowing why.

One Sentence

Recognize feel bad triggers.

Keep negativity out of the home.

Micro

You're out together, you're planning on having a great time :) you're there with your partner :) you're probably at a café, pressing your lips against your second cup of coffee dark roast, you've probably kicked your shoes off and your partner is scrolling/down/messages/on mobile :(This is called a micro date, not a *twogether* couple date. You're not maximizing time spent together.

If your partner is so busy txting to notice you; then what can you do except convince yourself that they are entitled to spend time txting, while you are pretending to be happy, who are you to be jealous of small things like electronic devices, who is this person they're talking to now, call waiting, take a message, send one anyway, sorry I've got to take this call, oh hi how are things. Who are you to complain? So you check out your mobile. That feels better.

"So listen, it's getting late... let's go?"

End of your so-so date! So digital. So cyber. So not sexy.

Seriously, turn off the phone. Turn off the electronics. It's a robotic anti-sex plot. Close down the mobile. Now you're ready to get down and get human. Geeks don't have as much real sex, cyber fact.

Micro

Spend time out together.

Leave your phone alone.

Neuron Buzz

When you fall in love, you have an above average level of endorphins and that's why you feel so incredibly happy with this incredible person. Everything feels positive until negative feelings start to creep in.

There is a negative and positive way to look at most things. If you feel negative, this doesn't create a sense of well-being for yourself or the people around you. So when you are feeling bad, don't make yourself feel worse by continuing negative thoughts on the subject. Talk yourself happy. You use an extremely powerful narcotic called thinking positively.

All you need on a daily basis to make yourself feel happy is to power up more endorphins! It's possible to do. If you use positive thinking as a narcotic, then the line of positive thought can produce a surge of endorphins. Tell yourself that you're in love with your work, in love with your friends, in love with that person you had an argument with. The thing is, your brain won't know the difference. By creating the illusion in your brain, the brain will believe it and you top up your endorphin levels.

Everything we do fires off neurons in the brain which release endorphins. How happy you feel, is dependent on the number of endorphins released into the bloodstream.

Take a bath and fire off 12 neurons, watch a great movie, fire off 69, read a French magazine 90, read Watermark by Joseph Brodsky 185, watch a butterfly 287, eat a smoked salmon bagel 320, a bowl of fettuccine 800, world famous Cirque 1530, lying in a hammock 2000, strumming a guitar 2205, snowboarding in fresh powder 3500, swimming in tropical blue water 4600, but an orgasm tops it all: millions and millions and millions and millions of neuron cells fire off in your brain!
Nothing can beat that!

Everyday problems can bring you down. So whenever a 'downer' issue comes up...counterbalance this by boosting natural endorphins through exercise, sex, a warm bath or shower, swimming, walking, massage, yoga and laughing. There are hundreds of ways to up your sense of wellbeing. Everything you do makes a difference to how you think. Everything you think makes a difference to how you feel.

Neuron Buzz

Be responsible for your own happiness.

Love Agendas

Let's look at the three most used words in the dictionary of lovers. I love you! It's easy to say. I love you. These words roll off your tongue. But notice how I love you, can come with certain conditions.

"I love you because..."

"I love you because you're strong."

"I love you because you're rich."

"I love you because you're sexy"

"I'll love you if..."

"I'll love you if you stay committed."

"I'll love you if you give me what I want."

"I'll love you if you stay attractive."

This kind of love is love that must meet and maintain certain conditions. Love becomes restricted and constrained within boundaries. The danger of conditional love is this. When someone more attractive, or more successful turns up, the conditional lover is really impressed. When you base love on conditions, and those conditions change, you'll be back looking for more conditional love. Then another chapter begins in the never-ending search for the perfect partner.

Partners who know they are loved for their strong points may be afraid to lose their looks or money or dance moves and spend all their time trying to keep up with expectations. They never let the partner see their vulnerable underbelly for fear of rejection. This lack of trust and inherent dishonesty affects the true potential of a long-lasting, loving relationship. Because, in the reality of life, all things change. True love is always unconditional.

Love Agendas

Keep your love unconditional.

Love is love is love.

I love you because... I love you.

Volcano

Imagine continuing to live with someone who thinks nothing of:

dropping a sulfur bomb

in the bed and laughing about it. Funny thing it's

not funny!

Someone who takes control of the TV remote, drops clothes, leaves dishes. Don't you hate annoying habits? So why do they insist on doing them?

Annoying habits are like an argument in mime. All action and no words. Then, if anyone does complain, they are accused of nagging! So what is really going on? If objectionable habits continue, even after you have highlighted them, there is an underlying problem. Annoyances are used as a form of dominate. Disguised as humorous antidotes or forgetfulness, annoying habits are used for power-playing the relationship.

Power-plays cause unspoken resentment. Eventually, a partner stops nagging and the annoyer thinks they are getting away with their actions. Not necessarily. For every action, there is a reaction. The annoyer ignores there is a tipping point. A point when the person living with them gets totally fed up with power play games. And then they withhold other things in the relationship to counter the power play. So if you're full of yourself, all gas, hot air, and sulfur, you'll end up being a right pain the ass and your love life will stink.

Volcano

Bad habits are not funny.

The Laws Of Desire

Ask someone who has been in a relationship for a while and you hear the same complaint. They never get enough sex. That's the biggest moan from men and women. They all say it's the partner's fault.

It's all up to you!
Take care of your physical appearance.

If you want to be sexy, you've got to feel sexy. If you want to be physically powered up. Who wants to go to bed with someone whose body odor reminds them of hamburger, fish & chips with vinegar or breath that has run out of mouthwash. It's sexual physics. When you were dating you made an effort to look attractive. So why stop now! Have a date night every week.

You know how to vamp things up. Here's the list to get physical: Improved diet and supplements, exercise, fresh air, showers, kissable breath, annual checks with dentist and doctor. You can buy new soap, aftershave, underwear, perfume, throw out the well-trodden socks. Buy brand new lingerie. Replace the tired and exhausted. Enroll in the gym again. Why not sign up and take some classes together! Rev up the endorphins, keep up the sweaty, sexy stuff.

Look in the mirror and check out the clothes you wear around your partner. Are you attracted to what you see? Relaxed casual does not mean slacking off and going into slob mode disguised as shabby chic! Look out for yourself and they'll be on the lookout for you!

The Laws Of Desire

Get physical.

If you want to be sexy, you've got to feel sexy.

Fireworks

Let's face it, you are two individuals with different opinions and points of view. You're going to see things differently and not agree on everything. But have you wondered how minor discussions turn into major conflicts so easily? How you both deal with a conflict of ideas or values, is where you get into fights.

Fights in themselves are not destructive things. How you handle the fighting is where you make or eventually break your relationship.

Fights are emotional fireworks.

Partners throw a few verbal crackers past each other. Let off a barrage of spinning incendiary thoughts, use searing sky-rockets to highlight unresolved issues. In the basic science of arguments, words and actions create uncensored explosions. Unchecked, small issues can be used as ammunition to get at your partner for all the myriad of ways they annoy you.

Right at the start of any disagreement you know if it's going to be more than a discussion. You will have recognized subtle body language, the manner, and tone of what's being said. The fight is in its infancy and you know it. At that point of knowing, you have to make a decision about which direction you want to go. Into the positive problem-solving discussion mode, or into the negative 'let's have this out now' battle stance.

Notice how often, you argue about small issues but there is also a dangerous undercurrent of unresolved issues that keep surging into the latest disagreement. Then your simple disagreement turns into an argument that rages out of control. Unresolved differences and grievances progress rapidly into a desire to slam the door on your intimate and physical relationship.

Who likes feeling less than perfect? Who doesn't take alarm at the first signs of blame? When it's pointed out that we are nothing less than infallible; we turn around and contradict, argue, justify, recriminate, rage, cry, do anything but give in to a partner who's pointed out your mistake. The real mistake is this: accumulating a dossier of issues and bad feelings may eventually shut the relationship down.

A relationship simply can't thrive on a constant litany of fights. Too much, too often and bad feelings erode the good feelings. So it's vital to be as emotionally generous as you can, especially if a fight is brewing: give up the blame game, maintain respect for each other, resolve conflicts by talking honestly and aim for a resolution in which each person understands the other's point of view.

Fireworks

Understand each other's point of view.

Avoid the blame game.

Don't accumulate a dossier of issues.

Love On The Bottom

Too busy and preoccupied to put lovemaking at the top of your list?

Take a look at what's going on. Are you facing more personal demands that impact on the time you have together? Has your workload increased? Are one or both of you working more? Do you have more bills to pay? Is life as demanding as it is overwhelming? Where is the fun in that?

OK, so let's say you are believers in each other and your relationship. That is a great start. To bring loving sex back into focus, try this; make a soft rule where you each get one night a week to say no thank you to having sex (for whatever reason you think of.) Then add in another soft option; as a couple, you can agree on a non-sex night. So two nights of no sex. Agreed. You get both nights off if you're tired or had an exhausting day. Now you're thinking how can having no sex increase your desire for each other. Well, what it means is, you're both guaranteed sex four nights a week if you desire! It allows you to see these as your special nights *twogether*. You can talk about ways to make those four days sexually orientated, such as showering together, having massages and everything intimate that makes you feel great as a couple.

And what about the days between? Make the most of all the moments: say goodbye with a kiss, hug and kiss each other every chance you get. Kissing keeps you connected. Make a point of connecting with your lover each day, no matter what is going on in your world.

Agree on a time every evening when you both stop your busy day. You can turn down the lights, light candles, play music. You are not trying to create a mood, by faking a romantic moment. You are just being together in the moment. Keep the sexual vibes going. Practice keeping the world out. The job, business, kids, friends, family, responsibilities, commitments and routine can impact negatively on your sex drive and intimacy. So take time to switch off the day and tune into each other. Avoid talking about problems for a while. Drink the wine and let the world be the world.

Love On The Bottom

Kiss, Hug. Love. Kiss. Hug. Love...Repeat!

Remember To Unfu*k Yourselves

Be a lover, not a leaver.

Agree to shake things up.

Bring issues out into the open.

Make each other aware.

Do a weekly emotional workout.

Be emotionally reliable.

Never threaten to quit.

Hurtful words do kill relationships.

Once you say something, you can't unsay it.

Love is a renewable resource.

Trust you can renew your relationship.

Commit to staying together.

Work through the bad patch.

Don't ruminate and fester bad feelings.

Do something good together.

Do something good for each other.

Keep a sense of humor.

Be patient with each other.

After an argument be close.

Maintain respect for each other.

Try to see each other's perspective.

Avoid being critical.

Avoid blaming.

Resolve issues sooner rather than later.

Get physically close.

Don't take negative behavior personally.

Avoid catching a negative mood.

Turn off negative thoughts.

Don't dump emotional trash.

Avoid being drawn into negative vibes.

Recognize your own negativity.

Say what's on your mind.

See your partner's point of view.

Jump the gap of misunderstandings.

Do something nice for each other.

Do the romantic.

Say the romantic.

Give the romantic.

Get communicating.

Be attentive and learn to listen.

Be supportive.

Don't ignore your partner.

Two ways. Your way and their way.

Respond to intuition.

Let spontaneity into your life.

Allow your partner to follow their intuition.

Equality rules.

Contribute to a love relationship physically, verbally and emotionally.

Listen more and interrupt less.

Give each other space.

Talk about how you're feeling.

Don't use moods as a weapon.

Don't cut your partner off.

Give each other time out.

Don't allow cyberspace to create space between you.

Make your bed a blah blah free zone.

Give each other verbal relief.

Keep your bedroom intimate.

Make your bedroom a discussion free zone.

Face and resolve daily issues that day.

Don't take unresolved issues to bed.

A peaceful mind makes sweet dreams.

Don't say what to do or how to do it.

Let your partner finish what they've started.

Agree on private codes between you.

Don't use a mood to manipulate.

Communication is an art form.

Express yourself.

Listen to what is said.

Equality does not weaken your partnership.

Create a balanced and equal relationship.

The silent treatment creates emotional stress.

A good listener makes a great lover.

Be generous in conversations.

Practice listening more and interrupting less.

Small talk brings you together.

Good communication is like emotional glue.

If you're flirting…then you're hurting.

Keep the real in relationship.

Stay in touch.

Build trust.

Be reliable.

Don't be secretive.

Don't be a freeloader.

Make individual decisions.

Share responsibilities.

Exchange responsibilities.

Give the respect you expect to get.

Talk as equals do.

Don't overlay past relationships onto this one.

See your partner as they are right now.

Be more of who you are, not less of yourself.

Don't block synchronicity.

Be an equal contributor.

Stop making your partner your body critic.

Pay each other compliments.

Your partner is doing it their way Let them!

Make individual choices.

Your partner has a right to personal choice. So do you.

Get interested and get involved.

Listen and speak the way a friend does.

Take time to be a good friend.

Get physically close.

Avoid being critical.

Give up the blame game.

Maintain respect for each other.

Try to see each other's perspectives.

Resolve whatever issue caused the argument.

Great communication creates greater intimacy.

Stimulate your relationship IQ.

Break out creative juices.

Make a commitment to stay together.

Do something about WeWe.

Avoid jealousy.

Be truthful.

Never lie...not even a white lie.

Don't tread eggshells around each other.

Don't screw up your relationship.

Do what you promise.

Do what you say you will.

Keep it *twogether.*

Great intimacy creates great passion.

Great love is within you both.

Blanshard & Blanshard

For Susan and Bruce, both students at the university, it was a love at first sight scenario. Six-months later, they moved into the upstairs of a rambling Victorian villa that had been converted into five doctors' consulting rooms. At 6 pm, when the doctors downstairs left for the day, Blanshard and Blanshard became the night cleaners. The rest is history. One by one, stuff got added into their life: a parrot, a stray cat, a vintage Jaguar, a baby boy, a baby girl, and along the way, busy careers.

Blanshard and Blanshard went on to become executive creative directors and bestselling authors. They are a creative team who share the same name and believe that a love can last a lifetime and it's worth everything to make it happen. Blanshard and Blanshard bring living and loving to their books. It's real relationship advice from a real couple who know what it takes to make a love last.

LOVE NOTES

A note from
Blanshard & Blanshard

Over the years, people have said things to us like: you two seem so happy together. What's your secret? Then someone sent us a note:

Happy Valentine's Day
Admired your love.
Wish when Dave and Me
get married we'll
be happy being together
like you guys.

It took that handwritten note to inspire us to write the book we'd been talking about for a couple of years. We wrote this book together because we believe in romantic everlasting love and being soul mates. Both of us take relationships seriously. Poets, artists, sculptors, musicians, mystics, philosophers have all waxed lyrical about the power of love. When you're in love, it's a powerful feeling, a natural magnetism, that is as dynamic as the earth's unending attraction to the moon. When you are in love, the best moments of your life are those spent together. Life is the two of you.

In the past, newly wed couples were given honey for the first month of their married life. Dining on honey was said to encourage love and fertility. If a relationship was as simple as feeding each other sweet stuff, that would be a buzz! But you can't just wing it. You've got to work at it. What we figured out is this. If you want to have a relationship full of passion and intimacy; a totally fulfilling relationship where you have great sex and feel sexy and stay in love; you've got to make it happen. The aim of the book is to share what we know, are ways to make love last forever.